POLLUTION SOLUTION CLIMATE RESTITUTION!

By Rose Marie B. Wolford-Zabala

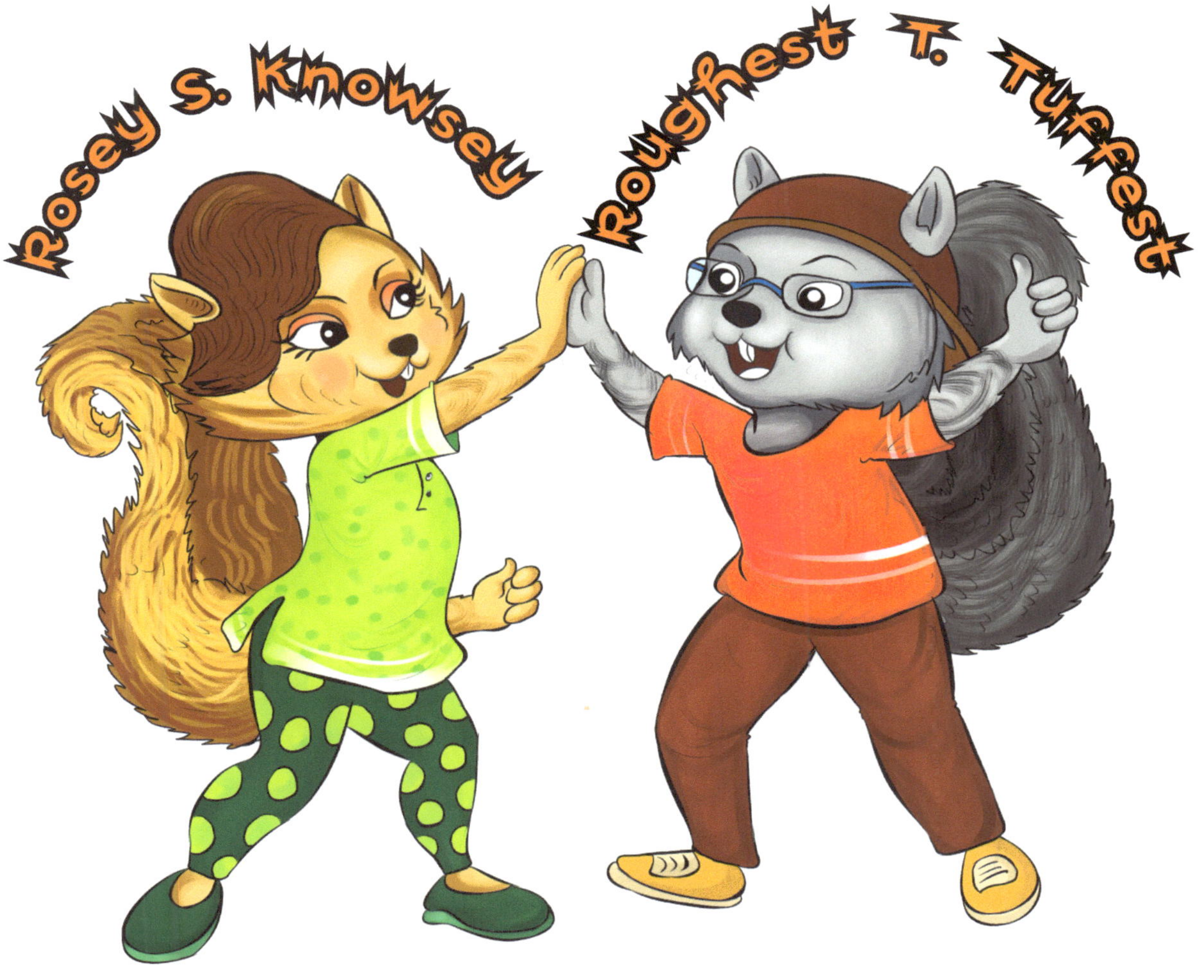

1

Rose Marie B. Wolford-Zabala

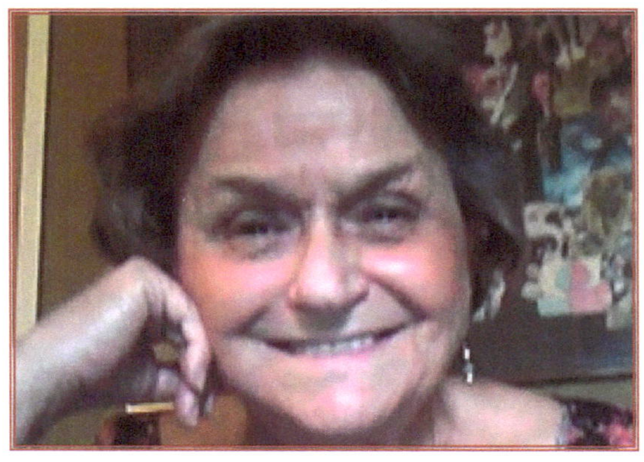

To the reader and 'read to' of this book:
Life is an ever changing energy
That resides inside of you and me!
If we take IT for granted and not protect IT
We begin to lose sight and to be apathetic!
The danger of this is the power we lose
To assure that our world is free from abuse.
The air and the water give LIFE, let IT flow
IT nurtures and cares, allows all to grow
For all living things need respect, care and honor
All have worth, having purpose ~ NONE to be just a fawner!
We simply CAN'T DENY IT ~ this RAPID CHANGE in CLIMATE!
To share a world together ~ respectfully in harmony
We must pledge to keep it clean ~ 'Clean and free protectors be'!

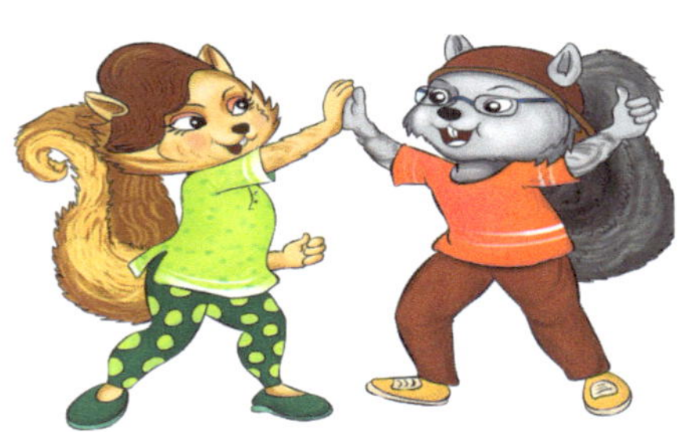

Special thanks to
Dolores (DD), French & Vilma Wolford

ISBN: 9798510718126
Carrie Campbell, Counselor/SUDCCII #6873, Palmdale, Ca. U.S.A.
Dr. Billy C. Lawrence, Theologian & Author, Colorado Springs, CO. U.S.A.
Susan Markebjer - Säfström, Behavioral/Counselor: Youth & Early Intervention,
Stockholm Vallentuna, Sweden
© Registration Number / Date: TXu001992006 / 2015-10-30

I'm grateful
to my parents
John and Katherine
Zabala who taught me
integrity. Many thanks to
my supportive endorsers who
believed in me and the subject
matters addressed in this book series.
Special thanks to my son Robb Wolford who
often encouraged and went through "huge"
amounts of collaborative and most likely often
frustrating editing. Thanks to all my sons and their
children . As well as, all the children who have always
inspired my spirit to keep on no matter what! And, of course
Father God, Who was and is and always will be I AM, that I AM

and
YHWH
for His
gifts
for
all

Special thanks to Shada Baduwi
who brought the characters alive in
the cooperative/collaborative efforts
illustrating and designing of this book:
ABC Education Materials and Training

Every once in awhile, we are blessed with beguiling smiling!
Thanks to my "relentless supportive fan, delightfully talented cousin Joann~
J. HERVANK…ENCOURAGE MECHANIC!

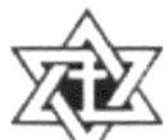

Faithful Father
Firmly Foretelling
Forever Fondly Forgiving
Fellows, Friends and Family
But let justice rundown like water.
And righteousness like a mighty stream
Amos
5:24

Rose Marie Wolford-Zabala is a Cognitive Behaviorist, Special Educator/Advocate and former Children Social Worker. Her experiences moved her to write the rhyming book series addressing current social-emotional, familial and environmental issues today experienced by families. At this point in time the third of 17 books to be published.

Rosey so Nosey and Roughest the Toughest series addressing:

Domestic Violence	Reading	Bullying
Divorce/Separation	Teamwork	Pollution/ Climate Change
Family and Global diversity	Hazards of Lying	Substance Abuse
Fear/Anxiety/Secrets	Stealing/Wrong conclusions	Water Conservation
Siblings fighting/reconciliation	Friends fighting and forgiving	Health Crisis/Safety

Rosey loved to explore and learn of "new things"

Not afraid of things different, while others did cling

To the same, not arrange, often shying from change

Due to fear of UNKNOWN and things out of range.

Rosey searched for the new and embraced this new treasure

Shared "discovers" with others for it brought her much pleasure

Roughest, her best friend helps find a way

Yes, they CAN find solutions and help save the day!

Let's all read together find what happened before

For the problem in store and we'll learn all the more

How Rosey and Roughest push problems away

Let's find out! All about…see what happened that day.

Roughest the Toughest **went out-NO delay,**
To go meet his friend for their
'squawk talk' that day.
Rosey so Nosey is quite a good friend!
He knocked on her door,
a greeting did send.
"Hello!" said Roughest to
Rosey's sweet mom.
She smiled down at Roughest
and **shared rather calm.**
"Dear Roughest I'm SO glad
you're Rosey's best friend but
she's so FRAIL and PALE...
indeed NEEDS to MEND.
So she can't leave and roam,
she's GOT to
STAY HOME!"

Roughest *SO*….disappointed,
asked Rosey's mom *"WHY?"*
She looked down at Roughest
and *let out a SIGH.*"Sometimes **our good air**
gets BAD THINGS *inside and for*
awhile... ITS
LOW TO THE SKY...
and when THIS happens
the good air will leave!

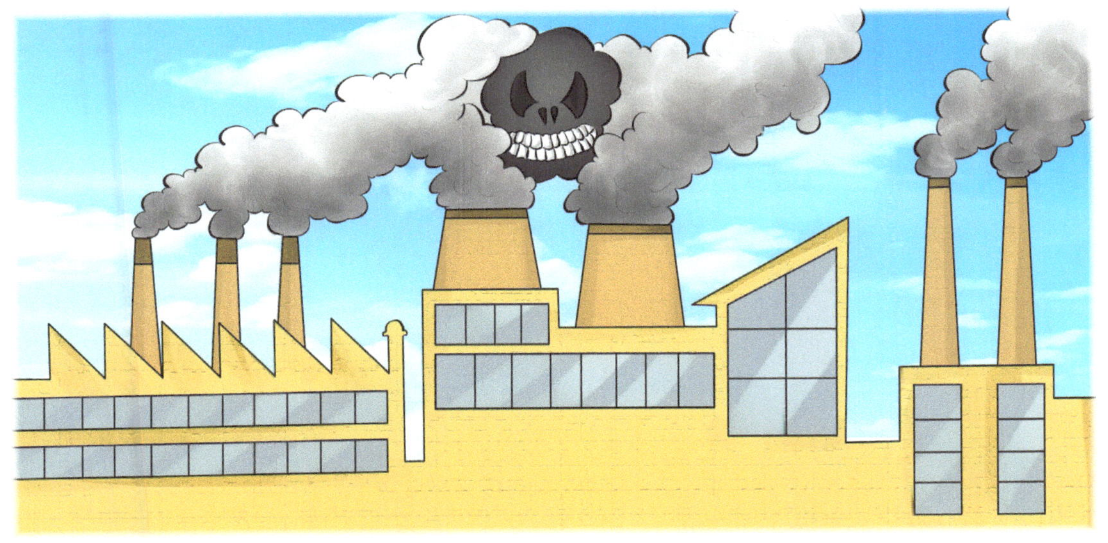

Folks just like Rosey...find it
SO HARD TO BREATHE!"

"Eyes get I T C H Y and D R Y
or watered with tears
ALL exposed CAN get sick....
young and old and all peers!
*Both the young and the old will
COUGH and will SNEEZE!*
All will hope that the wind can send
FORTH a B R E E Z E to BLOW AWAY

bad air so *GOOD* air C A N come!
TO *Replace* and *Restore* where the
BAD AIR *CAME* FROM!

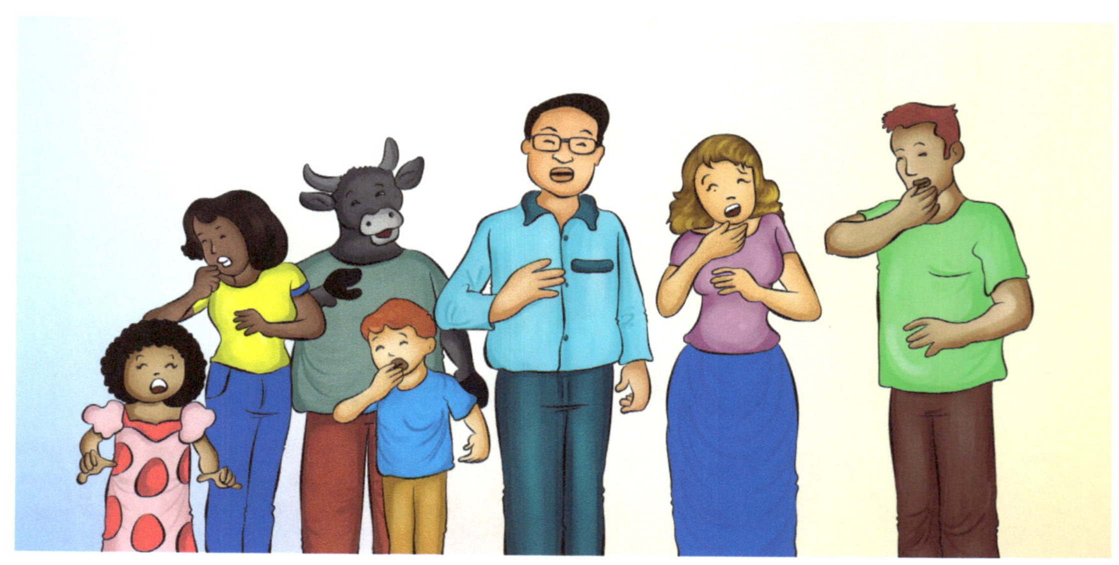

Rosey came down-
SUCH A FACE!   SUCH A FROWN!
Her eyes were all TEARFUL…her
BREATHING was down!
With a sigh said…"OH MY!
My H E A D and eyes HURT but HEY
good to see you SO glad you came by!" as

she SLUMPED with a SLOUCH!
Rosey 'C O U G H E D and
she S N E E Z E D' as she

PLOPPED on
the COUCH!

Her mom fluffed her pillow gave the blankets a tug. She smiled down at Rosey and gave a SNUG HUG!
Smiling up at dear Roughest said, *"Please use this chair,* for a bit you can sit, can visit *and share."* She left for the kitchen hurried back with a sack for Rosey and Roughest, a surprising good snack! Roughest felt OH SO SORRY for dear Rosey's TRIAL! He *missed her bright eyes,* her beguiling sweet smile!
Said, "Listen up Rosey- take care I'M RESOLVED! Pollution solution must be found! *I'M APPALLED!* That my dear friend *should suffer, many others* as well. We must ACT! It's a FACT! We must

SHOUT OUT
and TELL!"

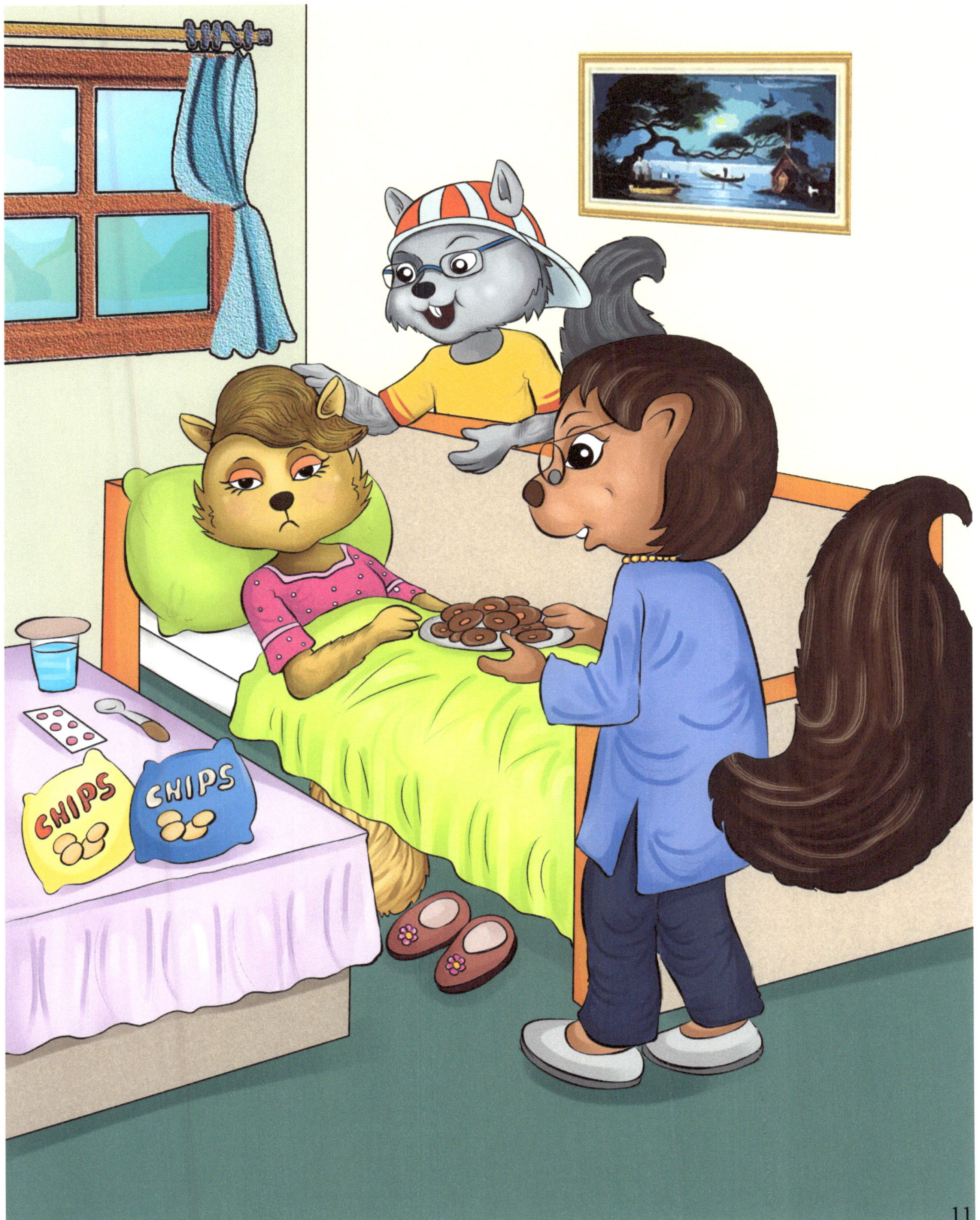
CHIPS
CHIPS

We must let others know! Make others AWARE! That we have a BIG problem- A Problem to Share! WE Need to take steps… ~^~^ 'BREED with SPEED' ^~^~^ MAKE SOLUTION! We JUST CAN'T sit by and ALLOW this POLLUTION! JUST CAN'T LET GO! GOT TO GO STOP THIS BLOW!

My father works with this! I've seen him chart it! I'll ask him to show us- we'll know how IT started! So then we can know how to crop IT to bop IT! To know how to

STOP IT!

RIGHT NOW...you CANNOT do...
what I'm certain YOU WOULD DO!
'YOU WOULD if YOU COULD'!
Let me get BACK to YOU!"

Roughest left!   When he got home he **didn't**
D R O N E he didn't M O A N!
He *yelped for help, yelled out,* "Hey Dad,
I'm really M A D and kind of SAD!
My good friend Rosey's **DOING BAD!**
I need HELP to find S O L U T I O N!!
Dad, I NEED and WANT to know–
I really 'NEED' for you to SHOW the
'Hows and Whys'...find RESTITUTION!
To stop the 'crimes that grind and
bind' PROMOTING this POLLUTION!"
His dad was glad and shared with him,
"We must make

RESOLUTION!"

"To *really CARE* for all earth's air… S T O P
FRIGHT, PLIGHT, FLIGHT! Beware and Dare!
Prepare, protect and stand against…
to be our GLOBAL WORLD'S DEFENSE!

Dad said sad, "THERE'S THOSE WHO POSE: 'There
is NO WORRY and THOSE 'WHO CARE' just cause
FLURRY! This trite 'CLIMATE WARMING WARNING'
Listen up, IT IS NOT forming! GOT TO STOP their
'scorning, mourning, storming global warning'!
Sometimes things just happen! IT'S NOT
SWARMING! Earth's resources aren't off course!
They're OKAY and here TO STAY!
There really are NO PROBLEMS HERE!
SO STOP this HYPE of GLOBAL WEAR!
No NEED to CHANGE so have NO FEAR!'
His dad pressed on with dread and said:
"By denying empirical data - supporting their
schemata…yet they've NO scientific proof just
S e l f - m a d e T H E O R Y :

SPOOF and POOF!"

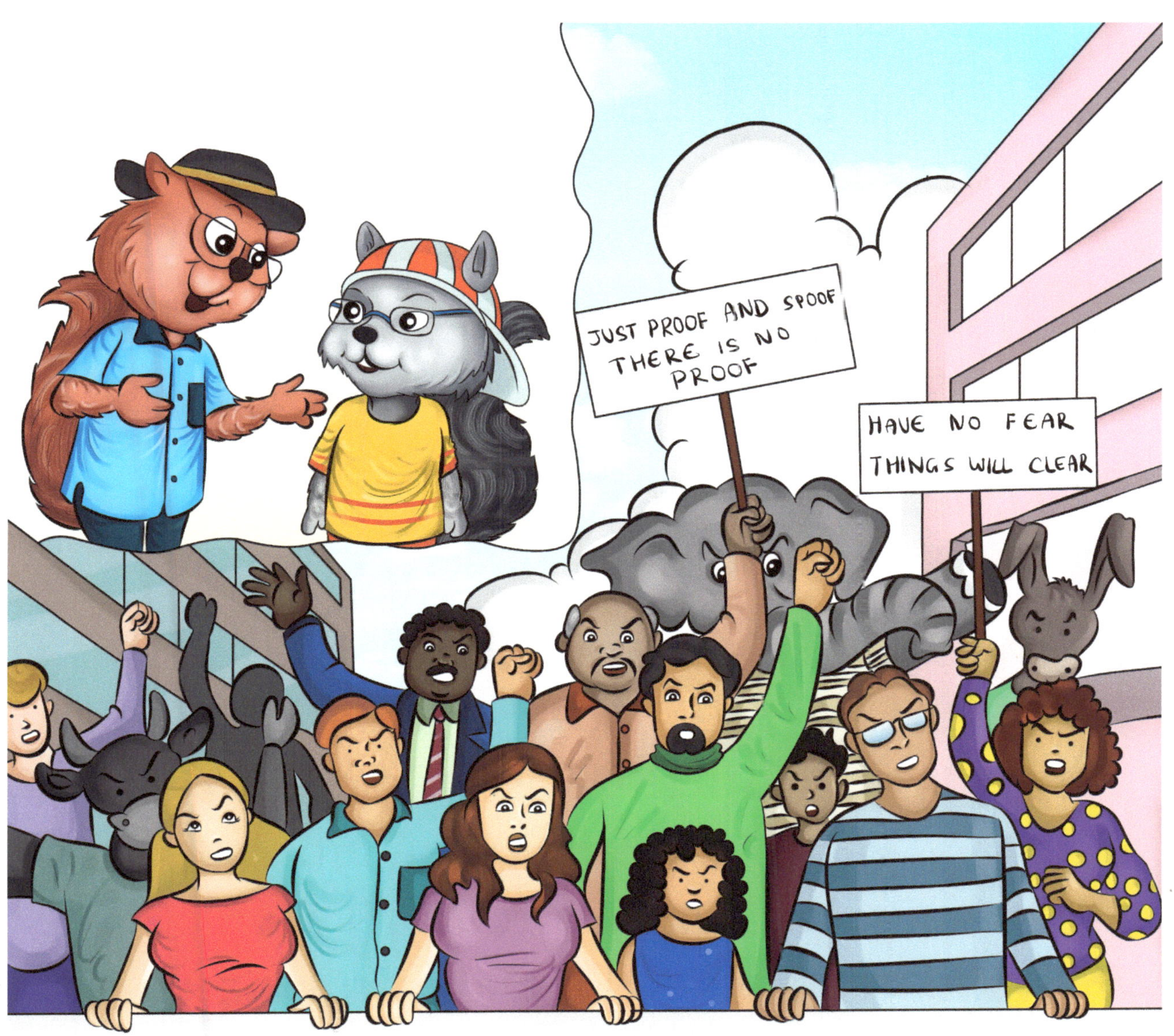

JUST PROOF AND SPOOF THERE IS NO PROOF
HAVE NO FEAR THINGS WILL CLEAR
GLOBAL WARMING ISN'T FORMING-
SO IT ISN'T SWARMING!

"Thinking so means *Jeopardy!*
DANGEROUS DISCREPANY! Those who
say, 'There's nothing wrong and strongly state
'NO RECOMPENSE!' Yet, GLOBAL HARM is
such ALARM! Such OFFENSE! No DEFENSE!"
Going on he said to Roughest...

"*One cause* is *the* smoke and soot that
CONTRIBUTE and REBOOT! *CLIMATE*
WARMING IS swarming! **And all of this IT**
will POLLUTE!   DISPUTE! CONFUTE!
Stand firm, impute! Be astute and resolute!
Cars and Factory's emission all promote bad
air transmission! Causing CLIMATE CHANGING!
Alarming-rearranging! Floods, fires, excessive
heat and cold! AS GLOBAL DAMAGES UNFOLD!
Truth be told-we must stand bold!
This horrid air that we all *share*
not fit for anyone to bear!
WE NEED to make IT STOP! BEWARE !
Need to dare! Need to C A R E!"

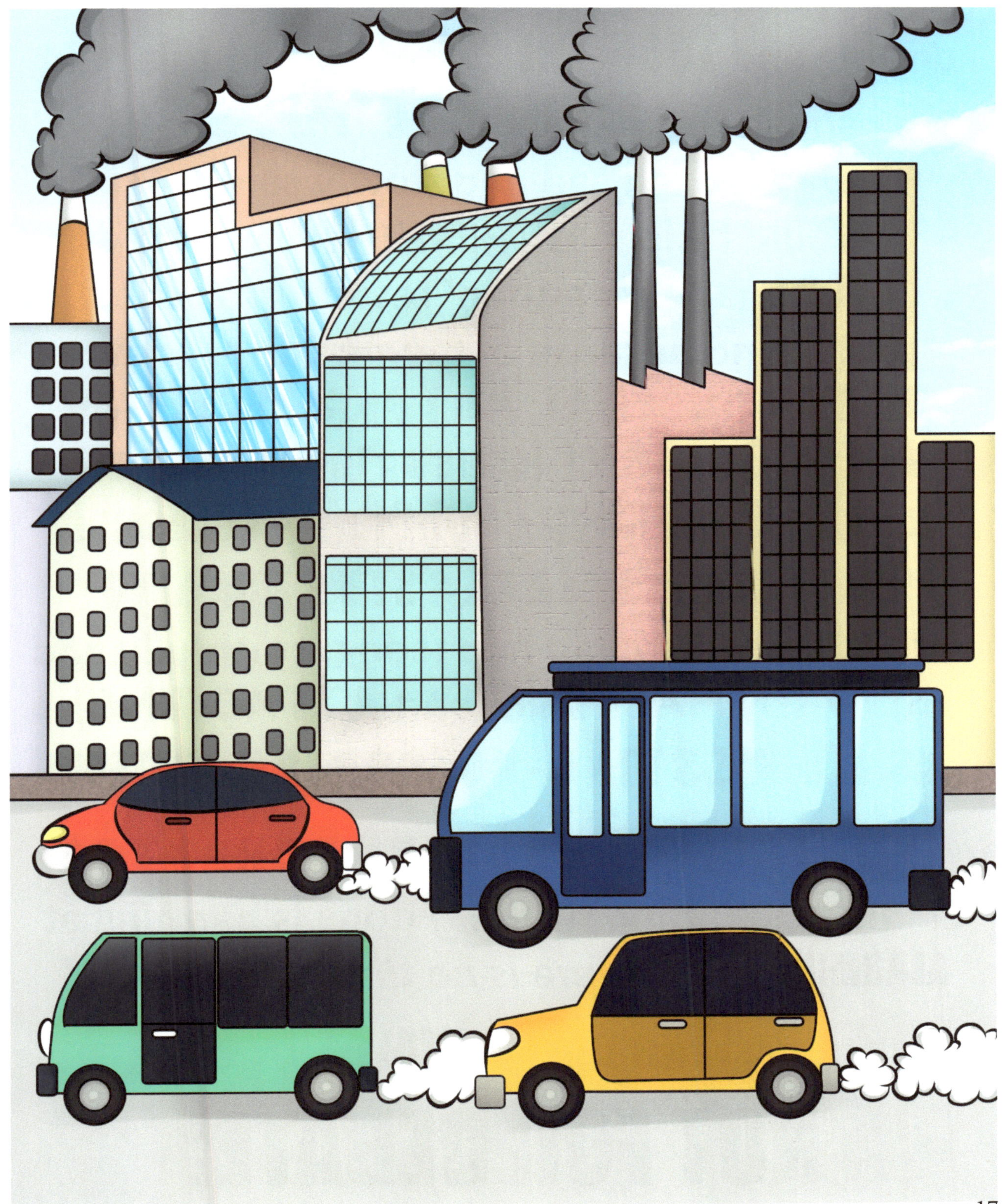

He asked, "Say, Dad **what if all** stopped driving and **TOOK THE BUS?** Would this help shush this '**CLIMATE FUSS?**"

His Dad looked sad and slowly said, "That would help but THERE'S **MORE** to **IT:** 'Caution to precaution' results in 'loss of profit' and because of monies hit 'they' **DON'T and WILL NOT do it! TOO MANY IDEOLOGIES** of industry technology-oft forego: **HYDROIogy – AGROIogy - ECOIogy!**

EXACTRACTING! EXCESSIVE FRACKING with ITS *cracking* and impacting, truthfully and ruthlessly HACKING and ATTACKING! **AS ITS WASTING-POISONING WATER!**

HONESTLY, IT SHOULDN'T OUGHT TO! *Drilling,* spilling, *killing* done is harming at **ALARMING** rate! There *is no time* to HESITATE!

NO TIME to WAIT...

NOT FOR DEBATE!

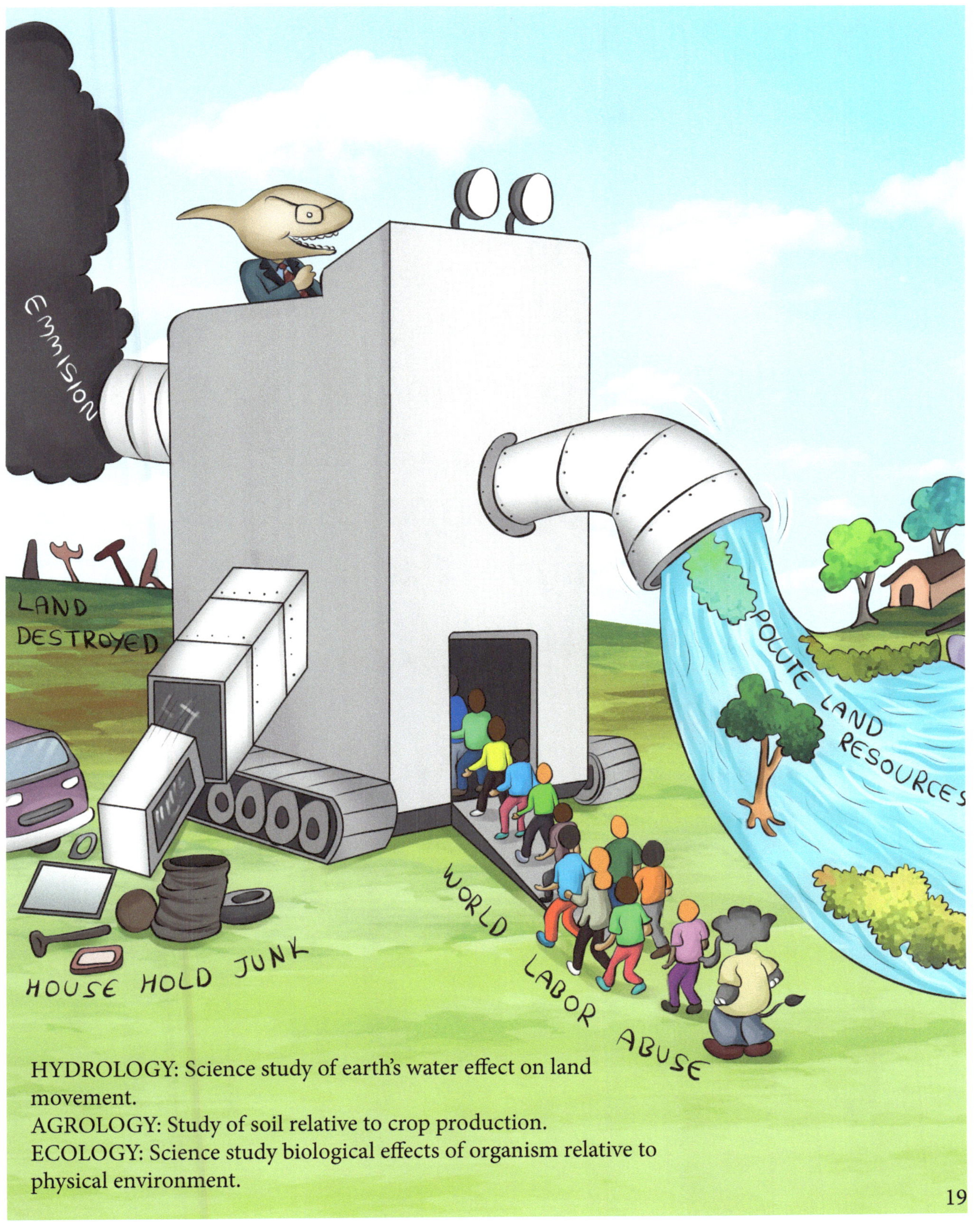

HYDROLOGY: Science study of earth's water effect on land movement.
AGROLOGY: Study of soil relative to crop production.
ECOLOGY: Science study biological effects of organism relative to physical environment.

"DRILLING DOWN throughout the ground, **SPIRALING-DIGGING** round and round! *Slowly changing* 'COURSE with FORCE'...going STRAIGHT- then to **THE SIDES** as IT streams and as IT glides... *As* 'chemical logarithms' permeate within **ITS SCHISMS!** Gases rising and dividing *throughout* the land -- *throughout* the air~

(DESPITE the BANS!)

while **Wreaking Havoc**

EVERY WHERE!"

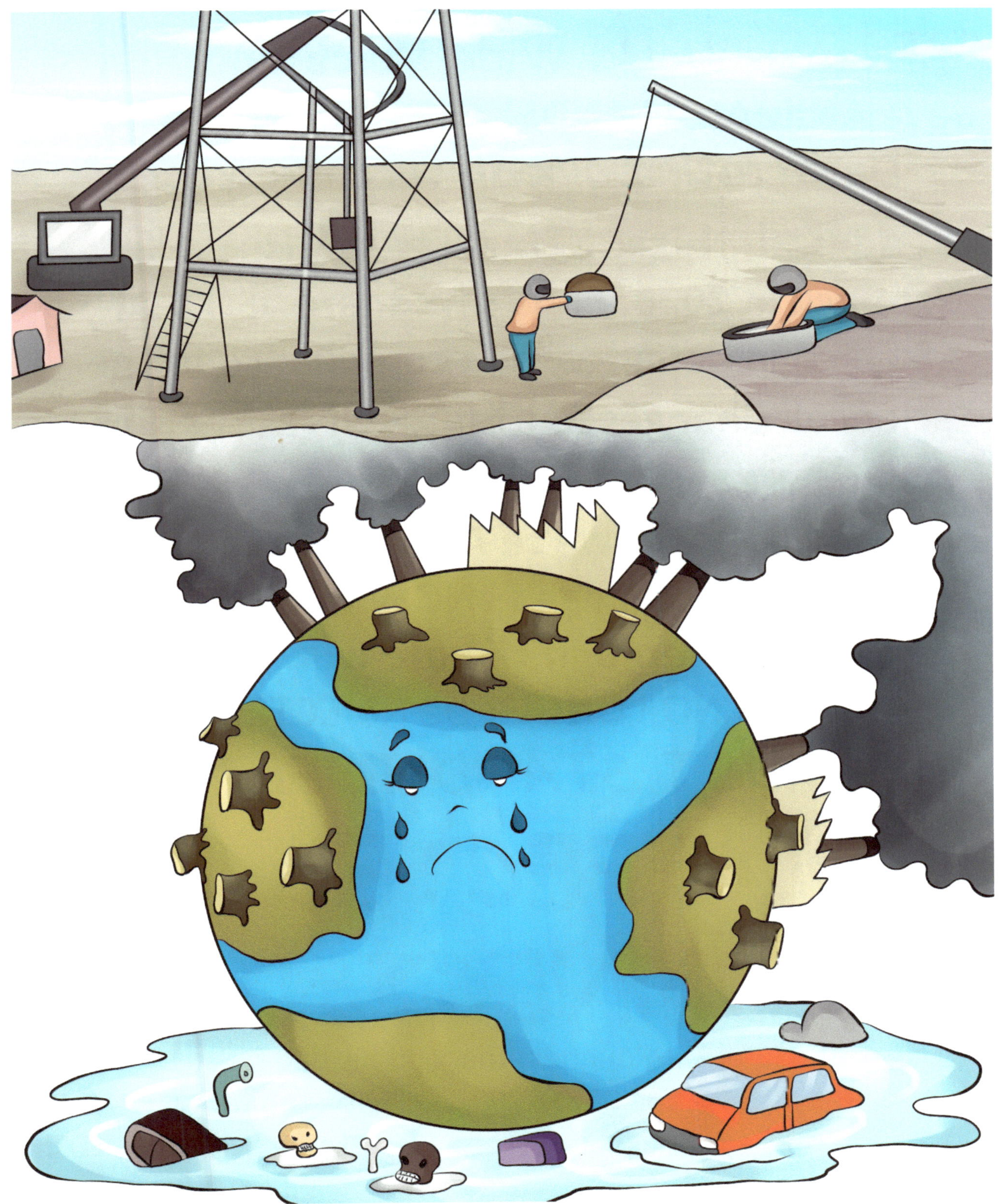

"IT causes World Wide Voice and Rants!
Save ANIMALS! LANDS! THE AIR! THE PLANTS!
Devastating global warming-years
denied this CLIMATE WARNING!
Yet back in 2020, Pres. says there 'ISN'T ANY!'
Said so in defiance, non compliance to the
science! Changes in ENVIRONMENT NO
longer CAN remain 'S I L E N T'!
GLOBALLY we're ALL AFFECTED.
Demand for change IS NOW EXPECTED!
Global storming climate warming...
CAN NO LONGER be REJECTED!
We MUST STAND TOGETHER
NOW! AFFECTED and
CONNECTED!"
Roughest thanked his dad for ALL he told:
Then *thought* 'I OUGHT
to be 'MORE BOLD'!

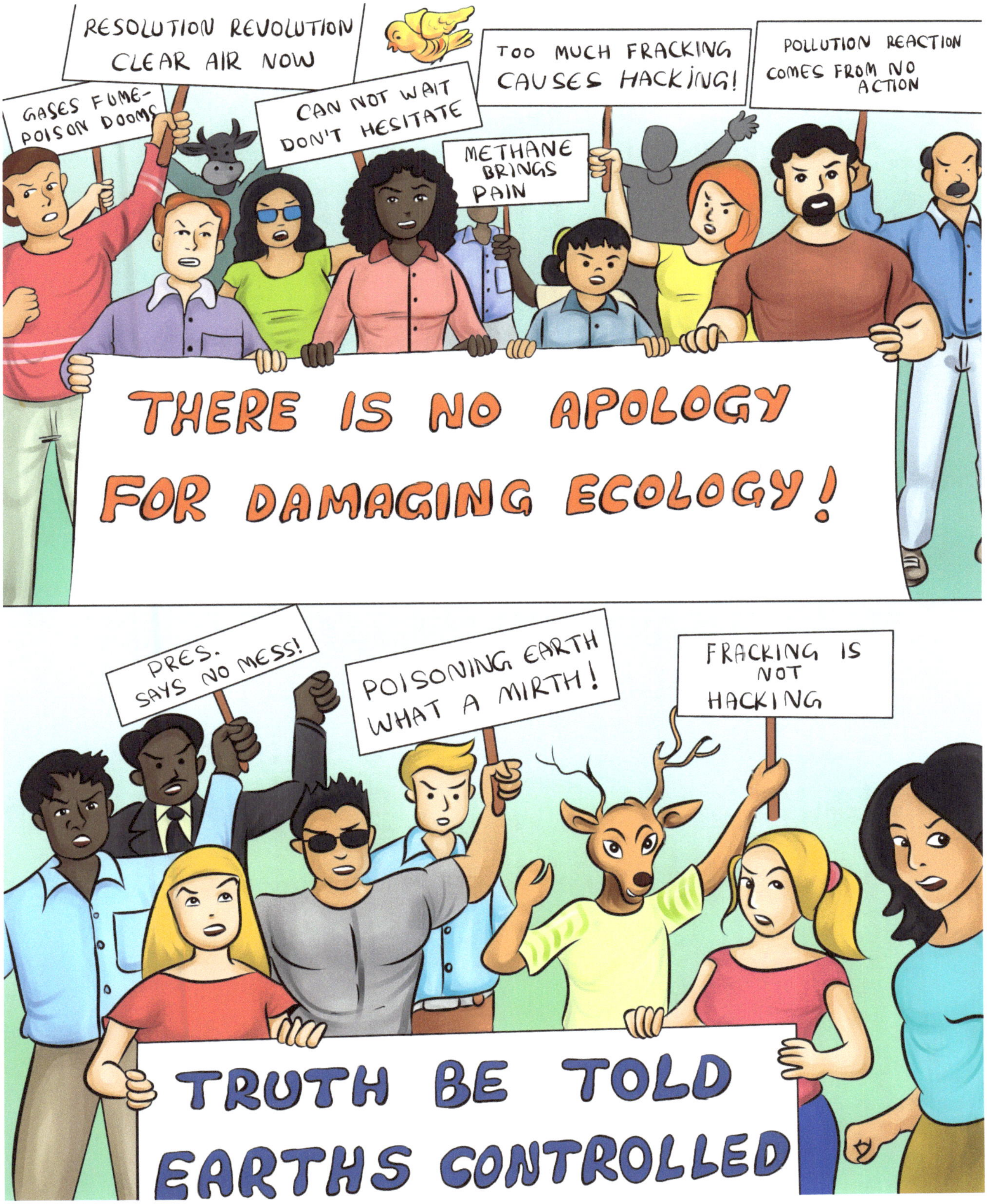

RESOLUTION REVOLUTION CLEAR AIR NOW
GASES FUME- POISON DOOMS
CAN NOT WAIT DON'T HESITATE
TOO MUCH FRACKING CAUSES HACKING!
POLLUTION REACTION COMES FROM NO ACTION
METHANE BRINGS PAIN
THERE IS NO APOLOGY FOR DAMAGING ECOLOGY!

PRES. SAYS NO MESS!
POISONING EARTH WHAT A MIRTH!
FRACKING IS NOT HACKING
TRUTH BE TOLD EARTHS CONTROLLED

He told all to Rosey while playing a game. "When YOU'RE FEELING *bet*ter we'll **SHOUT OUT OUR AIM!**" Rosey agreed said, "**YES, INDEED!** There surely **IS an AWESOME NEED! THIS WE SHOULD SPOUT! ALL SHOUT OUT ABOUT… THIS ZAPPINING HAPPENING** and what we 'CAN DO'! TOGETHER ENSUE BAD AIR *to SHOO*! So FRESH CLEAN AIR IT CAN get *through!* We'll 'veer to steer' a HULLABALOO! Clean our air and help **RENEW!** Let's do it with a BALLYHOO! All of us! Me and you! Bid BAD AIR FAIR FOND *ADIEU!*"

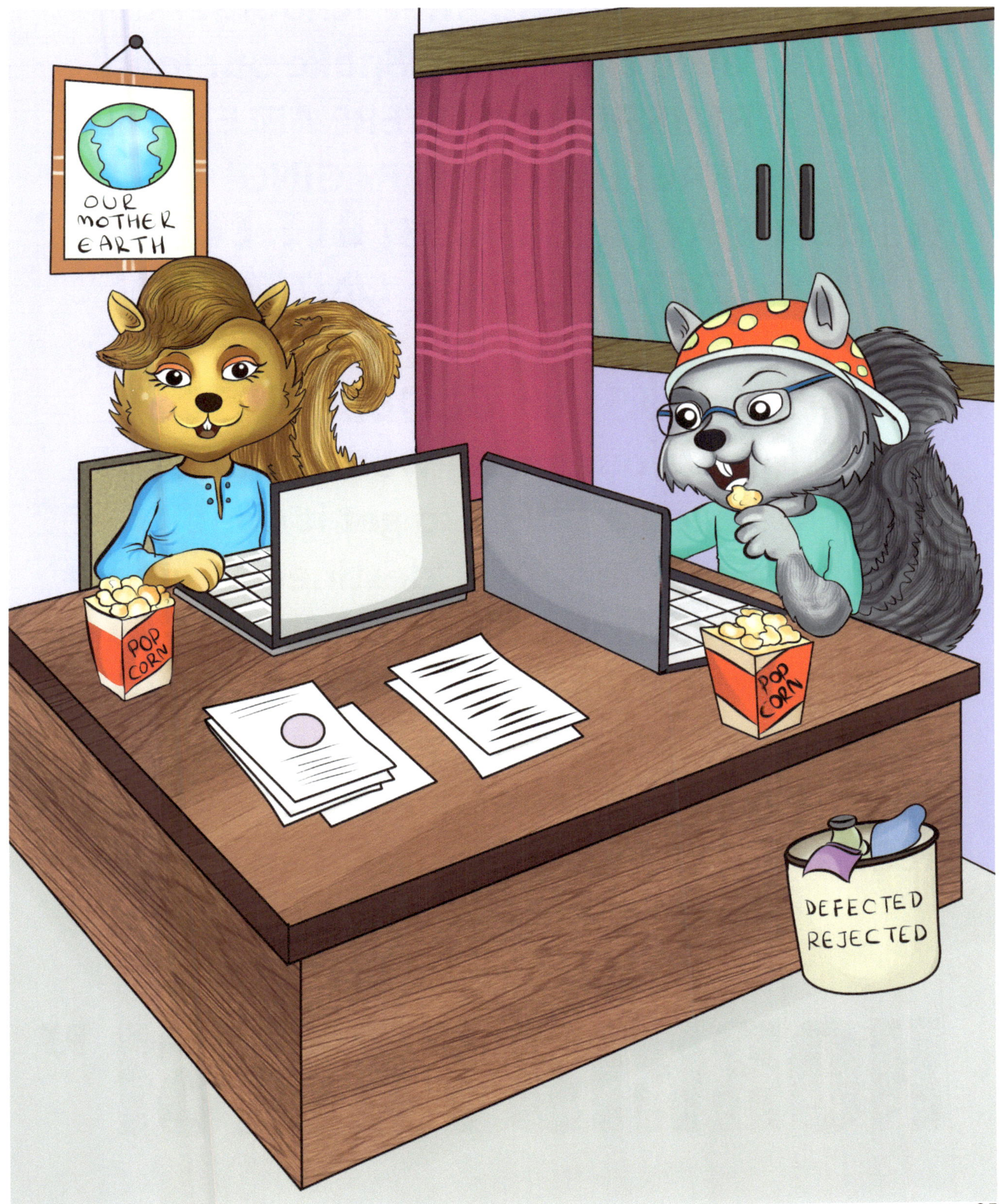

OUR MOTHER EARTH
POP CORN
POP CORN
DEFECTED REJECTED

Rosey and Roughest, after school set up a
table. Faced the crowd! Spoke out loud!
Had PERMISSION and WERE ABLE! "This
TRAGEDY'S DISPARAGING!
We can't STAY CALM! MUST **GET EXCITED!**
Be IGNITED! Be UNITED!
FIGHT for RIGHT! YES, *SIDE* BY *SIDE!*
ALL of US for GLOBLE PRIDE!
To save our global world as one
we need a **CREED** to get it done!
Future generations ARE 'destined *to inherit*`
an earth of little worth! **Unflt to Grit-SO we
CAN bear it! NOT fit a bit for us to share it!**
A world *'stripped of resources'* from
'too long known forces'! A world that can't
REGENERATE! That suffocates! Can't hesitate!
Climate change IT cannot wait!
DEFLATE to GATE these

HORRID FATES! "

COME JOIN THE FIGHT TO MAKE THINGS RIGHT
OUR WORLD IS SUFFOCATING
WE'VE GOT TO
STOP THIS WAITING !

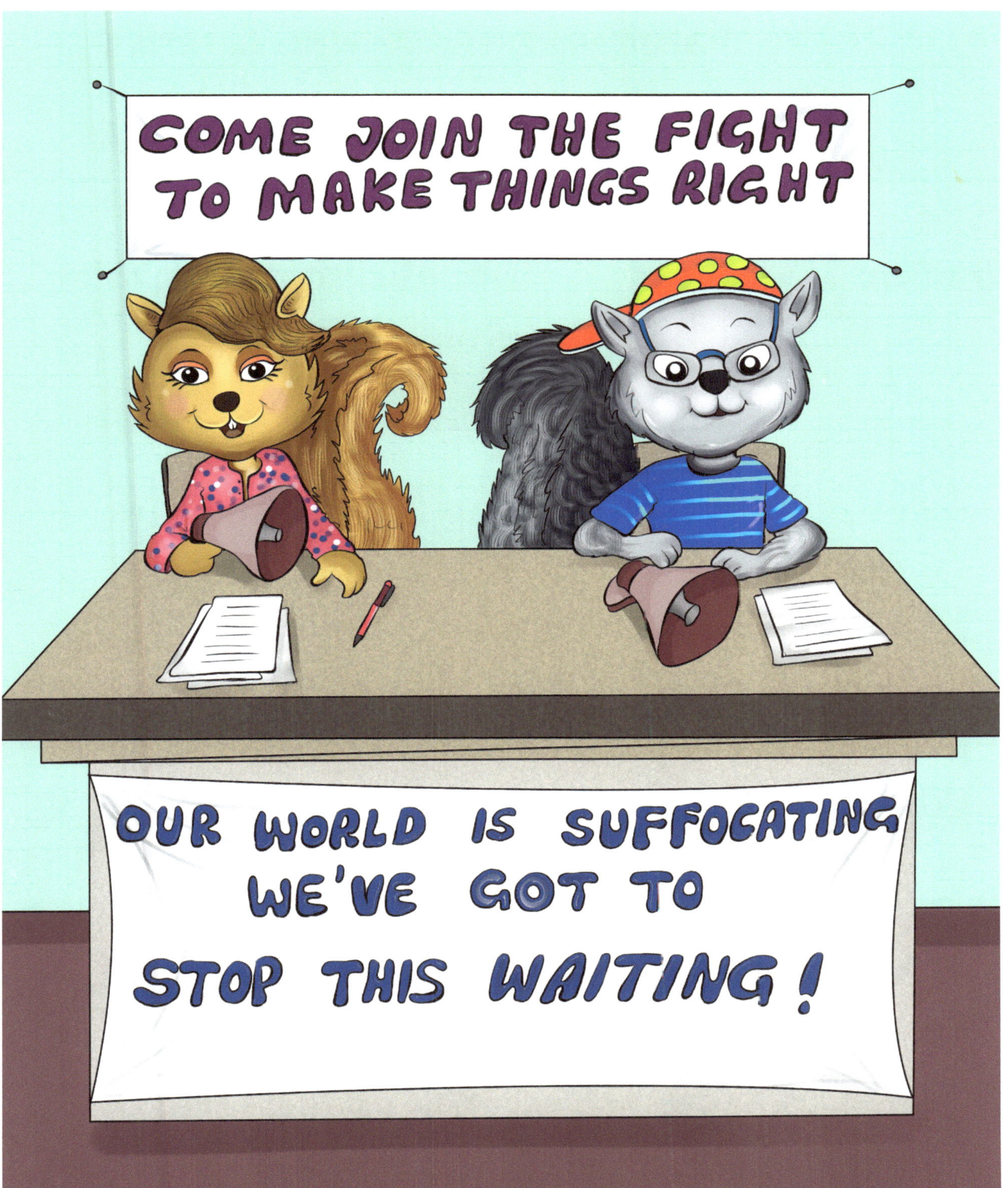

27

Rosey shared with those who cared:
*"There was a 'teen girl' years ago
who shouted out... to make* **IT** *known.
She is a Swede and yes indeed...***IT** *still goes on
and on* **ITS G R O W N!** Global climate warming!
ITS warning on while swarming!"

~~*~*~ READERS!* **Join Rosey and Roughest! SAY with me! SO folks will see!** *~*~*~*~*

Let's shout **IT** out! Bring **IT** up! Stir **IT** up!
Get **IT** done! Earthquakes shaking!
Fires breaking! Tsunamis waking! Icebergs
MELTING! Harm RESULTING! Species living
in 'THESE PLACES' **HABITATS A T T A C K E D!**
While climate change *DISOLVES-ERASES!*
It is a fact! We've got to act! IF NOT they'll
have NO PLACE TO GO! Earth created
long ago- intent with natural balances. **Y E T**
destroying, exploiting - stripping and ripping

G O E S on 'without' ANALYSIS !
ATTACKS and cause PARALYSIS!

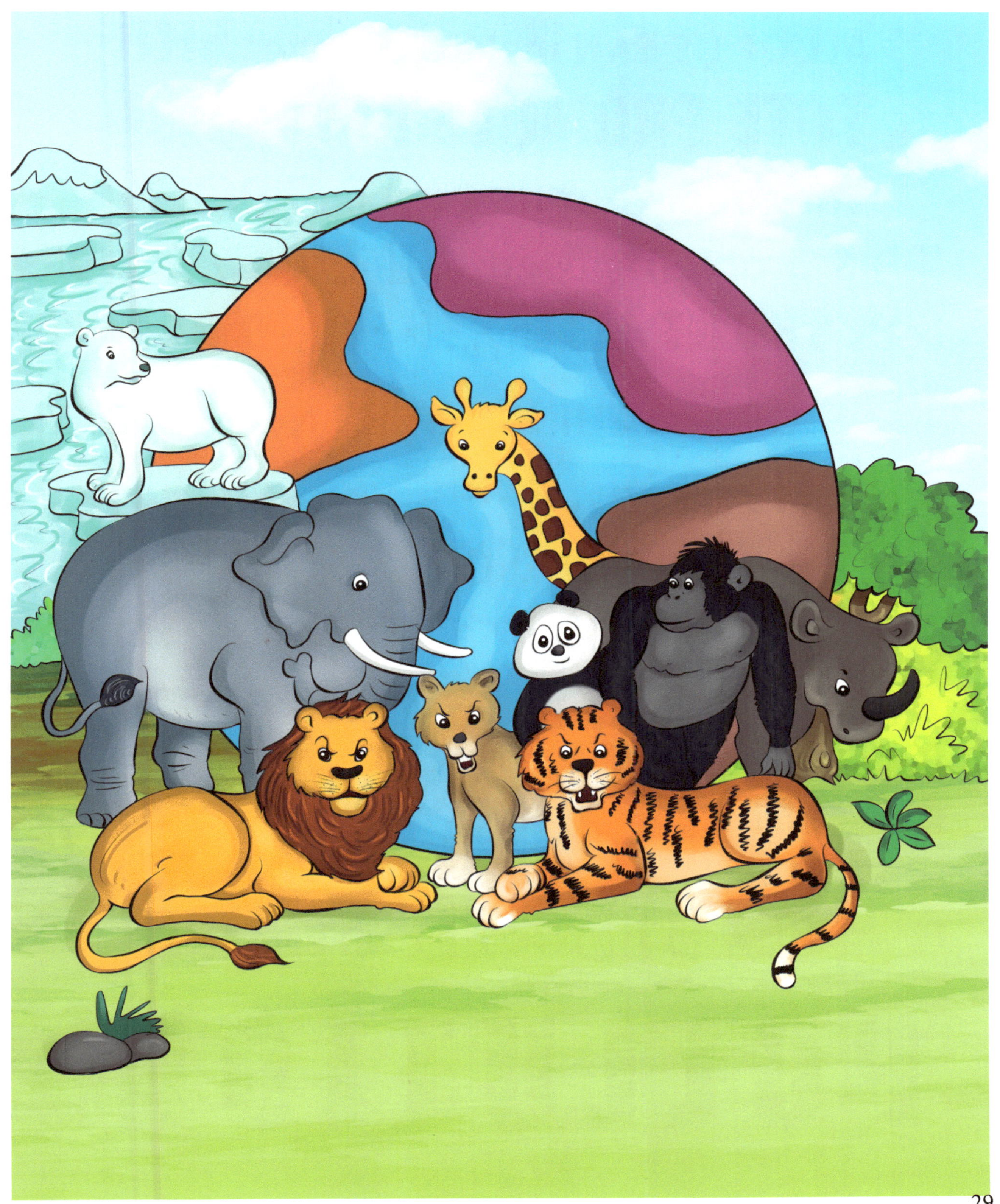

ALL OF US CAN make a change...**HELP**

TOTE PROMOTE AIR FLOW!

Loss of air- it is *NOT GOOD!*

This problem posed *WILL* only grow!

Let's **SHOUT** and say... **HEY! NO DELAY!**

Let's STOP and THINK! RIGHT NOW TODAY:

Restitution -~- Evolution!

GOT to FIND SOLUTION!

ALL make *CONTRIBUTION!*

START A

CLIMATE REVOLUTION!

'TO BID RID' of this

POLLUTION!

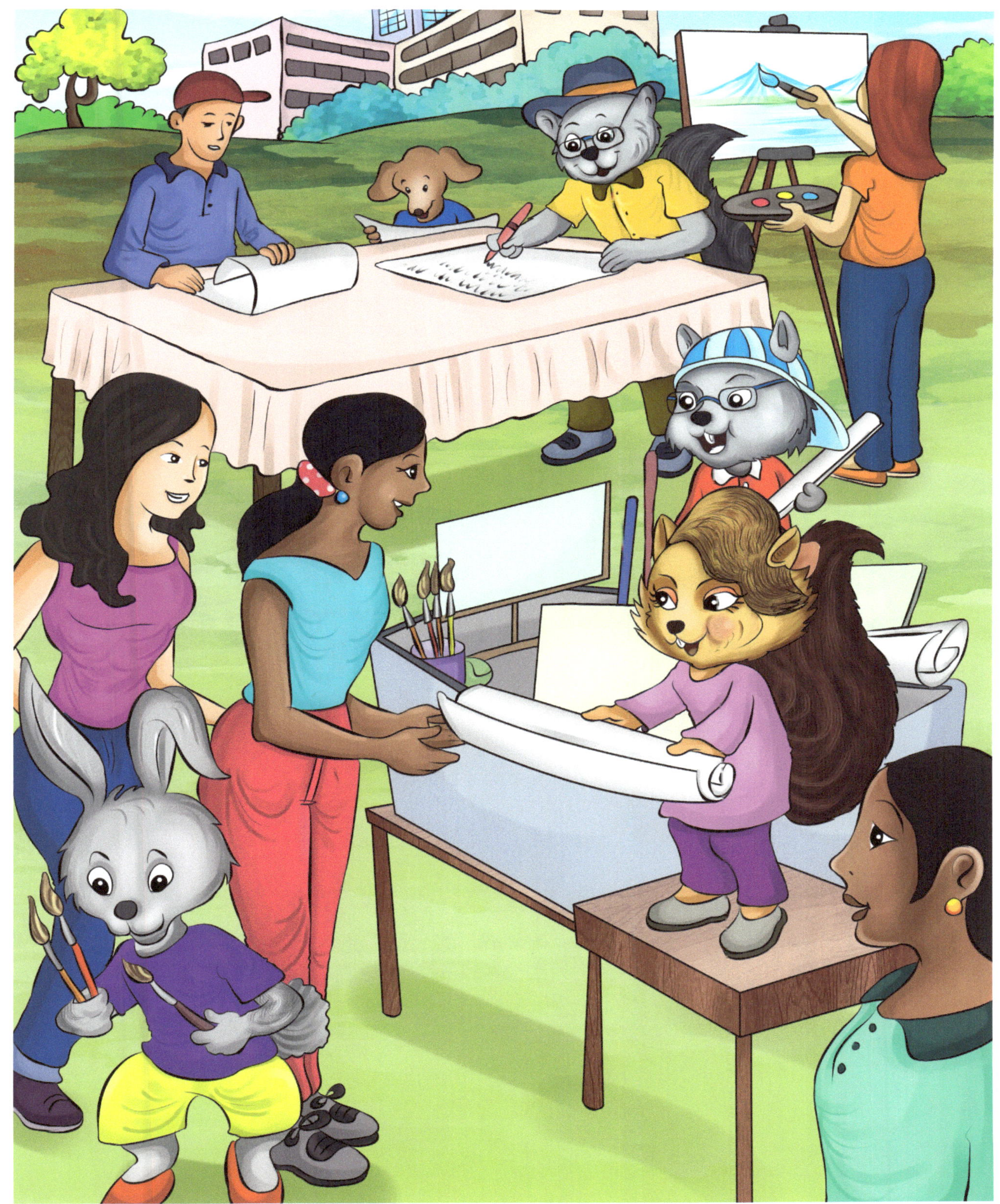

**PUT DOWN YOUR IDEAS!
TALK THEM UP!** DARE to 'CARE and
SHARE' with others... we're all
GLOBAL SISTERS, BROTHERS!
We need 'good air' to BREATHE
and W I N D S *to HELP CLEAR!*

Cannot Shush! We *must* Rush! Got to Crush!
THIS BAD AIR ITS got to VEER!
Cause a BLOW! OPPOSE *ITS FLOW!*

That taunts and haunts
while *bringing* FEAR!
To young and old...
to *flowers and plants... from the*
L A R G E S T of C R E A T U R E S
to the t i n y s m a l l a n t s !

GOOD AIR! Giving the Living
so **OUR** whole world **CAN** grow!
Let's get started TODAY!
START RIGHT NOW! HELP IT *FLOW!*
Ask *friends*! Ask *strangers*! Ask *adults*!
When asking ALL- no 'insult results'!
`YELL!` `Give YELP!` `GO GET HELP!`
We cannot stall....this continuous
genesis *perilous* call'!

We must thwart
this climate morph!

DON'T be BOUND! ASK AROUND!
Tout with clout! Bout and *SHOUT!*
WHAT *CAN HAPPEN? -IF NOT?*`
IF *SOLUTIONS* aren't *FOUND?*

IF SOLUTIONS...

NOT SOUGHT?

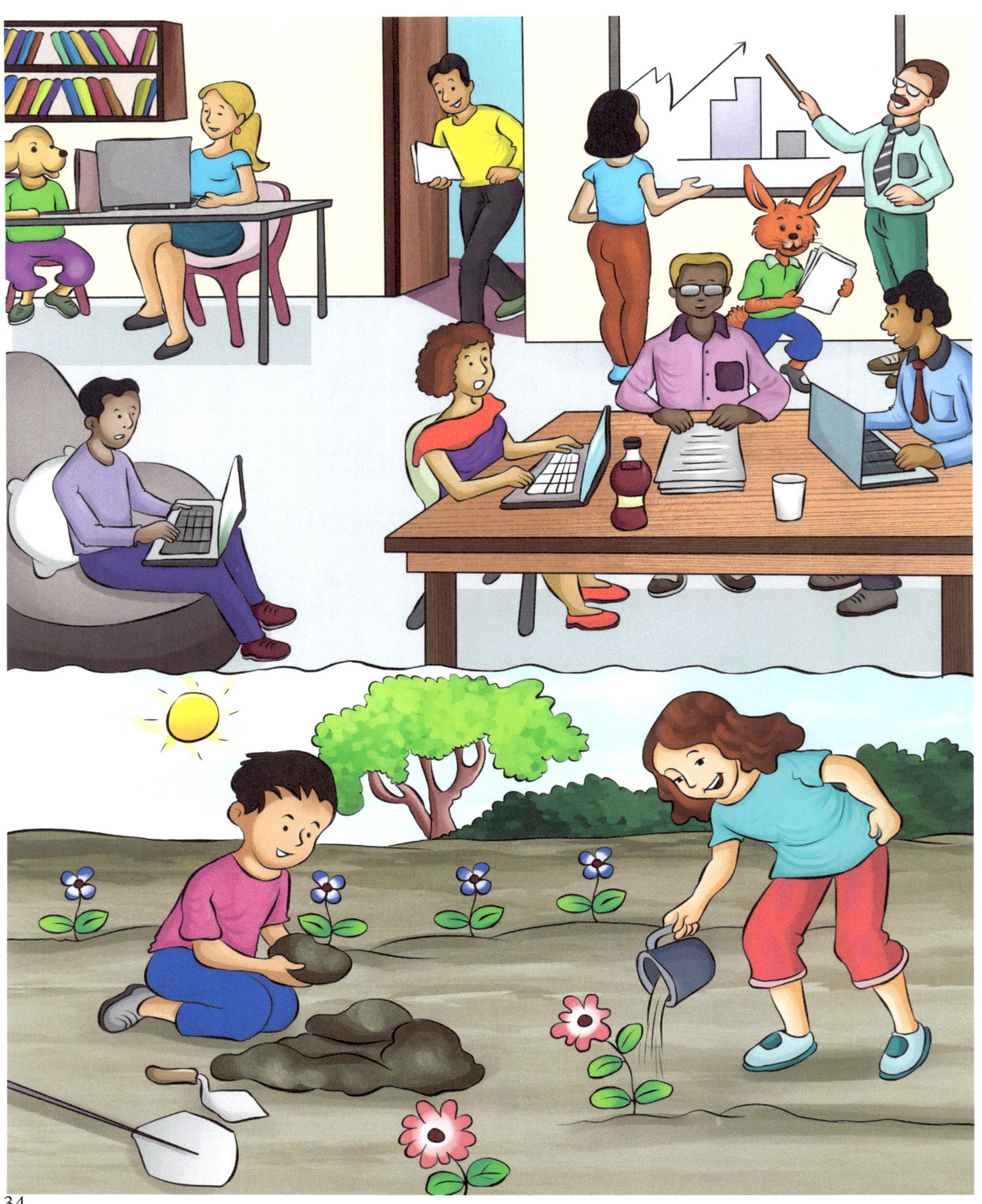

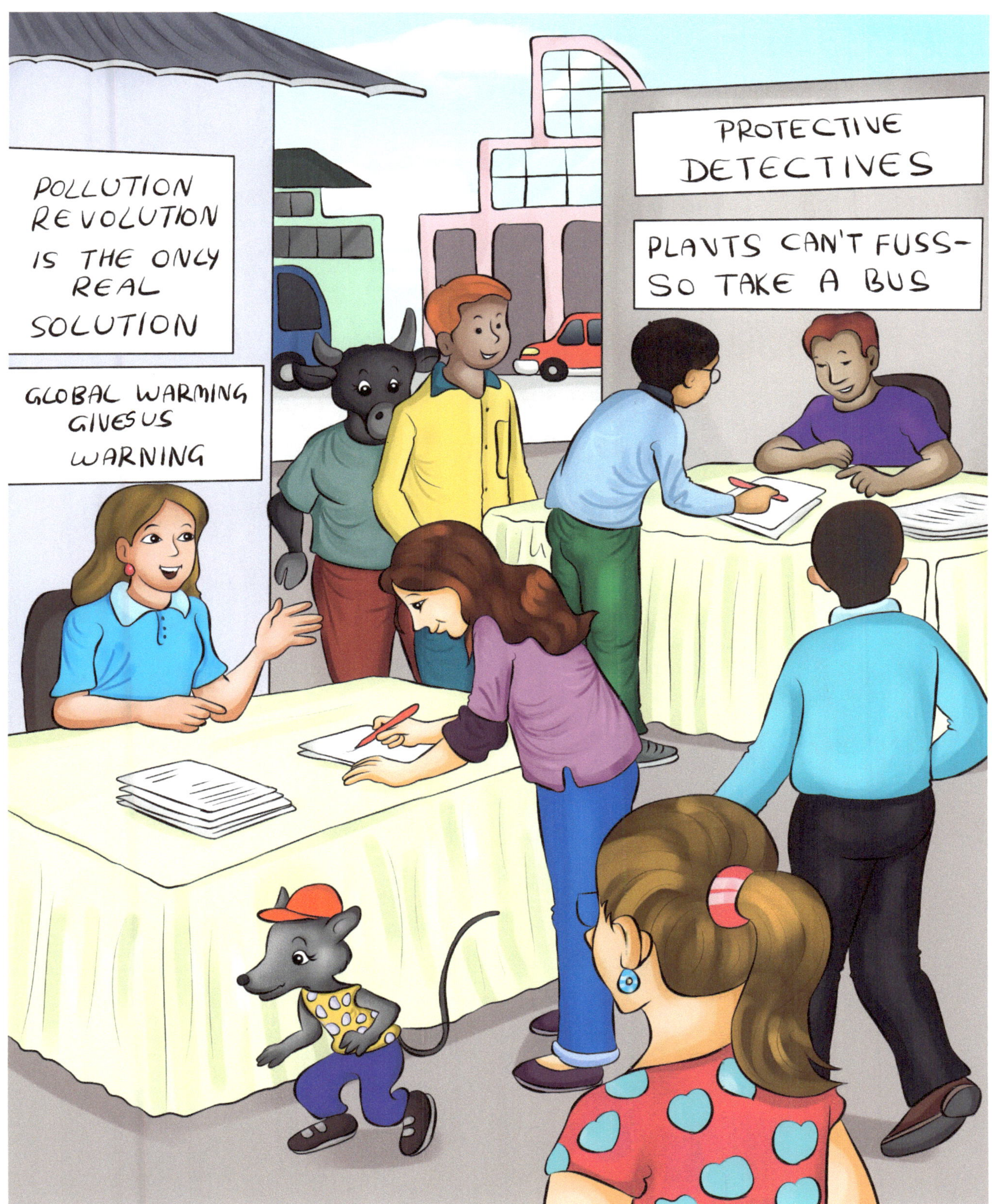

POLLUTION REVOLUTION IS THE ONLY REAL SOLUTION
GLOBAL WARMING GIVES US WARNING
PROTECTIVE DETECTIVES
PLANTS CAN'T FUSS— SO TAKE A BUS

TOGETHER NOW!
'DARE TO SHARE!'

Find out ways 'TO' clear the air!

Do you have some thoughts?

Thoughts, you'd like to share?

EFFECTING WATER, LAND and AIR?

STOP the 'lethal gain' ... of growing

CLIMATE CHANGE!

CANNOT STALL! Rise up BOLD!

Rise up TALL! HEED the call! SAVE us ALL!

Time to 'ROOT and BOOT' this

NEEDED INSTITUTION...

RESTITUTION

EVOLUTION!

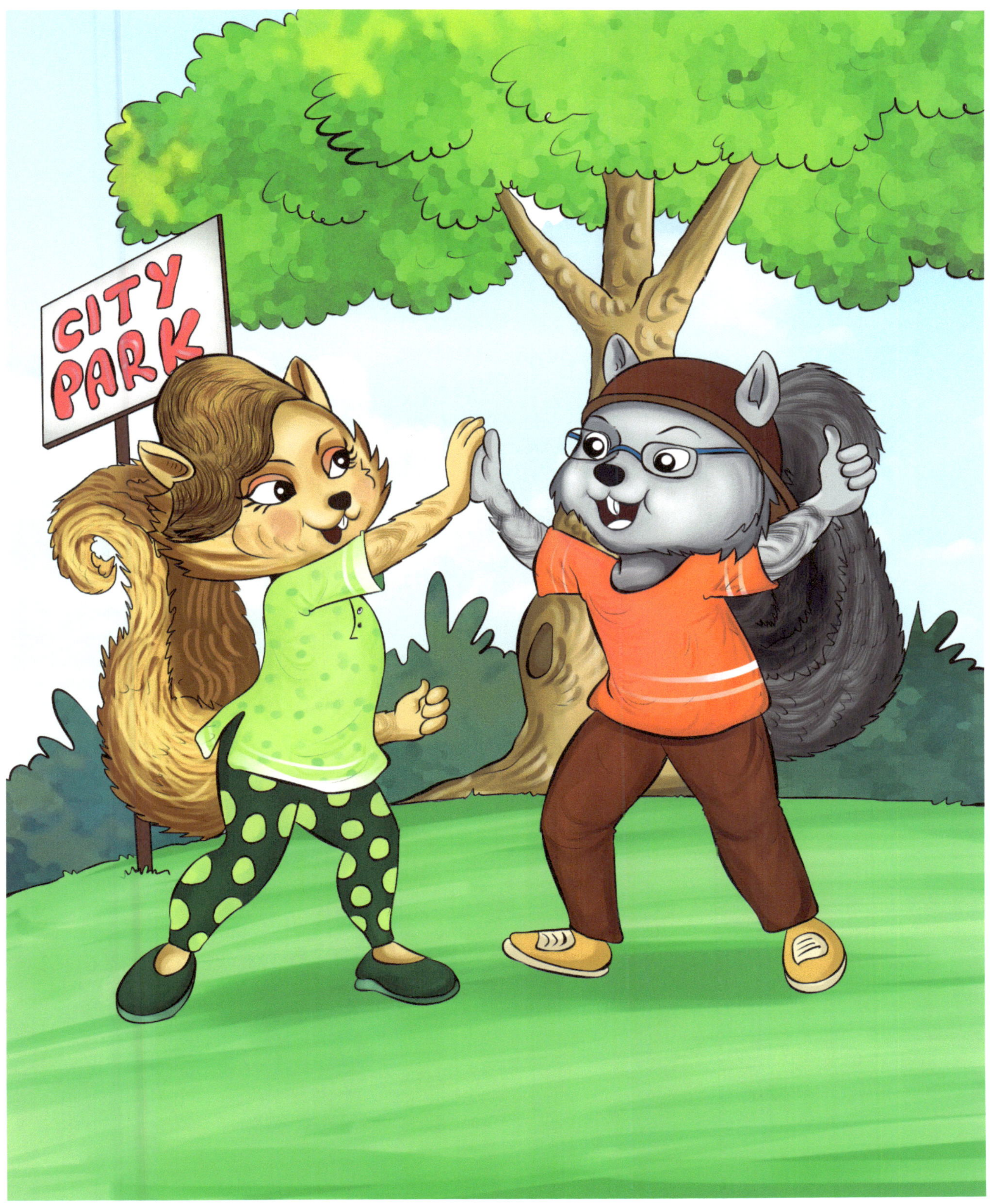
CITY
PARK

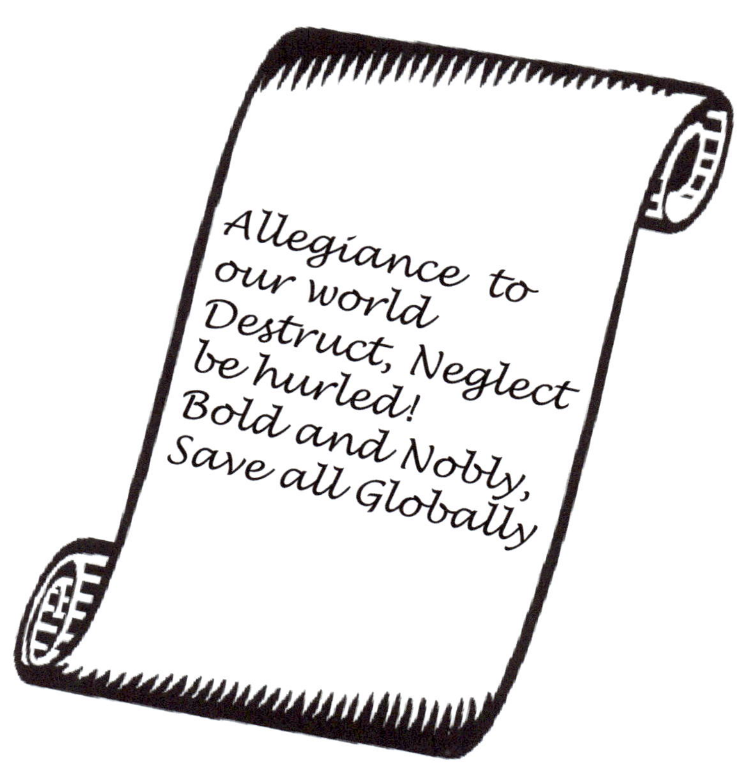

Our whole 'PLANET'S ON EDGE'   GO AHEAD! MAKE your PLEDGE!
Do what YOU CAN DO! SAVE our WORLD and HELP RENEW!
Mandala "pledge to save our earth" available by contacting climate
activist J. Hervanek bopeep007@gmail.com)